Cumulative Record/Practical Record for Basic B.Sc. (Nursing) Course

(NTR University of Health Sciences, Vijayawada, Andhra Pradesh)

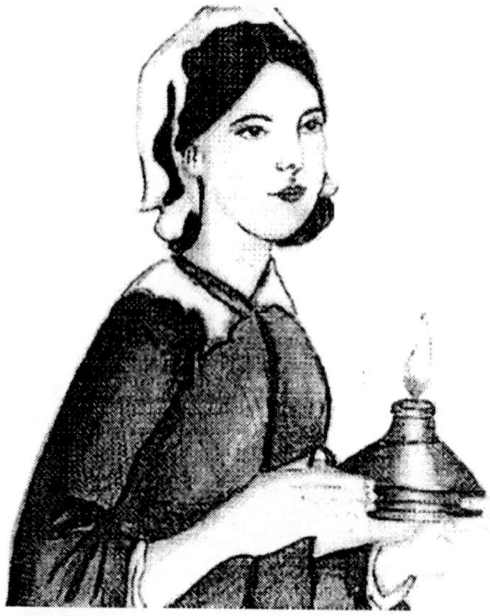

...MISS FLORENCE NIGHTINGALE...
PIONEER OF MODERN NURSING

Born on: 12th May, 1820

Died on: 13th Aug, 1910

The Nightingale Pledge

I solemnly pledge myself before God
and in the presence of this assembly
to pass my life in purity
to practice my profession faithfully
and to maintain at all times
the highest standards of nursing care
and of professional conduct
I will respect the religious beliefs of my client
and will hold in confidence
all personal information and family affairs entrusted to me
I will carry out the physician's orders
intelligently and loyally
I will abstain from whatever is deleterious and
mischievous and will not take or knowingly
administer any harmful drug
I will devote myself to the welfare of those
committed to my care
I will adhere to the standards of personal and professional ethics
which will reflect credit upon my profession
I will do my utmost
to fulfill the fundamental responsibility of a nurse
which is four-fold
    To promote and to maintain health
    To prevent illness
    To restore health
    and to alleviate suffering

Cumulative Record/Practical Record for Basic B.Sc. (Nursing) Course

(NTR University of Health Sciences, Vijayawada, Andhra Pradesh)

As per INC Revised Syllabus 2012-2013

Third Edition

KP Neeraja
MSc (N) MA BPR PhD
Professor of Nursing
Channapatna
Karnataka, India

Jaypee Brothers Medical Publishers (P) Ltd

New Delhi • London • Philadelphia • Panama

Jaypee Brothers Medical Publishers (P) Ltd

Headquarters

Jaypee Brothers Medical Publishers (P) Ltd
4838/24, Ansari Road, Daryaganj
New Delhi-110 002, India
Phone: +91-11-43574357
Fax: +91-11-43574314
Email: jaypee@jaypeebrothers.com

Overseas Offices

J.P. Medical Ltd
83 Victoria Street, London
SW1H 0HW (UK)
Phone: +44-2031708910
Fax: +02-03-0086180
Email: info@jpmedpub.com

Jaypee-Highlights Medical Publishers Inc.
City of Knowledge, Bld. 237, Clayton
Panama City, Panama
Phone: + 507-301-0496
Fax: + 507-301-0499
Email: cservice@jphmedical.com

Jaypee Brothers Medical Publishers Ltd
The Bourse
111 South Independence Mall East
Suite 835, Philadelphia, PA 19106, USA
Phone: + 267-519-9789
Email: joe.rusko@jaypeebrothers.com

Jaypee Brothers Medical Publishers (P) Ltd
17/1-B Babar Road, Block-B, Shaymali
Mohammadpur, Dhaka-1207
Bangladesh
Mobile: +08801912003485
Email: jaypeedhaka@gmail.com

Jaypee Brothers Medical Publishers (P) Ltd
Shorakhute, Kathmandu
Nepal
Phone: +00977-9841528578
Email: jaypee.nepal@gmail.com

Website: www.jaypeebrothers.com
Website: www.jaypeedigital.com

Inquiries for bulk sales may be solicited at: jaypee@jaypeebrothers.com

Cumulative Record/Practical Record for Basic B.Sc. (Nursing) Course

First Edition: 2007
Second Edition: 2008
Third Edition: ***2013***

ISBN 978-93-5090-422-0

Printed at Replika Press Pvt. Ltd.

Dedicated to

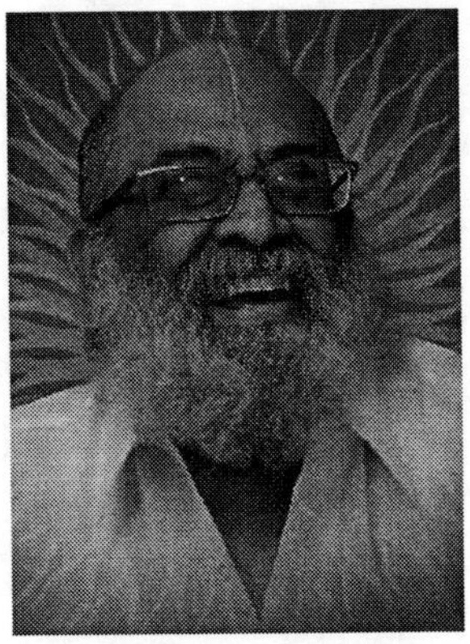

My Spiritual Father
Poojya Sri Sridhar Guruji

Student Record

Name of the Student : ....

Date of birth : ....

Age in years : ....

Educational qualification : ....

Father's name : ....

Residential address : ....

....

....

Name of the Institution : ....

Place : ....

Reg.No. of Student : ....

Date of joining into B.Sc. (N) course : ....

Date of completion of B.Sc. (N) course : ....

Identification marks : 1 ....

2 ....

Signature of the Student

Date:

Signature of the Principal

Date:

Guidelines to use the Cumulative Record

The clinical record is a teaching aid, is prepared as per the syllabus of NTR University of Health Sciences, Vijayawada, Andhra Pradesh, 7th Publication (July 2012 -2013). This record would provide the information regarding the practical experience gained by the student nurse under strict clinical supervision during the course.

The clinical supervisor/teacher will give instruction about purposes of procedure, steps to be carried out during the procedure, care of the equipment after the procedure and demonstrate the procedure in lab. After return demonstration in both lab and in clinical area satisfactorily, the student is allowed to carry out the procedures independently in clinical settings. It ensures that the nursing procedures learnt systematically by the student during training. Academic year wise the procedures that are learnt by the student in all the specialities, are listed out. Entries has to be made immediately after the procedure with due care. The student should show keen interest voluntarily and obtain signature from the clinical supervisor. Concurrent evaluation is performed to assess the clinical performance of the student. The Cumulative Record will be submitted to the University Examiners at the time of final practical examination of each subject, for scrutiny.

KP Neeraja

I Year B.Sc. Nursing—Hours of Instruction

Name of the Student ....

Reg. No. ....

Total Hours: 1480

Sl No	Subjects	Theory (in hours) (Class room and Lab)	Practical/Clinical Hours	In Hours	Name of the Subject Teacher
1	English	60	–	–	
2	Anatomy	60	–	–	
3	Physiology	60	–	–	
4	Nutrition	60	–	–	
5	Biochemistry	30	–	–	
6	Nursing Foundations	265 + 200	450	–	
7	Psychology	60	–	–	
8	Microbiology	60	–	–	
9	Introduction to Computers	45	–	–	
10	Hindi/Regional Language	30	–	–	
11	Library Work/Self-study	–	–	50	
12	Co-curricular Activities	–	–	50	
	Total Hours	**930**	**450**	**100**	

Attendance of the Student (%) :

Theory :

Practical :

Character and Conduct :

Extra-Curricular Activities :

Co-Curricular Activities :

Signature of the Class Coordinator
Date:

Signature of the Principal
Date:

I Year—Scheme of Examination

Name of the Student ....
Reg. No. ....

Month and Year of Passing:

Sl No	Subjects	Duration of Exam in Hours		IA Marks				Marks in University Exam				Total marks		Month and Year of Passing
				Theory		Practical		Theory		Practical				
		Theory	Practical	Max marks	Marks obta-ined	Max marks	Marks obta-ined	Max marks	Marks obta-ined	Max marks	Marks obta-ined	Total marks	Total Marks obta-ined	
1	Anatomy and Physiology	3	–	25		–	–	75		–	–	100		
2	Nutrition and Biochemistry	3	–	25		–	–	75		–	–	100		
3	Nursing Foundations	3	3	25		100		75		100		T: 100 P: 200 Total: 300	T: P: Total:	
4	Psychology	3	–	25		–	–	75		–	–	100		
5	Micro-biology	3	–	25		–	–	75		–	–	100		
6	English*	3	–	25		–	–	75		–	–	100		
7	Introduction to Computers	3	–	25		–	–	75 (school exam)		–	–	100		

*English: Passing mark – 40%

- Distinction – 75% and above; I Division – 60% to 74%; II Division – 50% to 59%, Pass – 50% (Theory – 50%, Practical/Orals/Viva put together – 50%).
- 5 attempts is permitted to pass each subject; If the student failed in more than 2 subjects he/she will be detained in the same class; If 1 or 2 subjects failed, the candidate will be promoted to the next class.

Signature of the Class Coordinator
Date:

Signature of the Principal
Date:

NURSING FOUNDATIONS

Sl No	Name of the procedure	Date of demo in lab	Supervisor's signature	Date of clinical return demonstration	Clinical Supervisor signature
1	**Hand wash technique**				
	Utilizes medical and surgical aseptic technique				
2	**Coat technique**				
3	**Preparation of clients' unit**				
	Disinfecting clients' unit				
	Bed making				
	Unoccupied bed/open bed				
	Occupied bed				
	Special beds				
	Preoperative bed				
	Cardiac bed				
	Fowler bed				
	Orthopedic bed				
	Postoperative bed				
	Amputation bed				
	Burns bed				
4	**Utilizes effective communication methods by utilizing the skills** – Attending skills				
	– Rapport building skills				
	– Empathy skills				
5	**Establishes therapeutic nurse-patient relationship and professional relationship**				
6	**Admission procedure**				
	Emergency admission				
	Routine admission				
	Transfer-in				
7	**Documentation and Reporting**				
	Maintains records and registers				
	Admission register				
	Nurses notes				
	MLC record				
	Linen book				
	Diet book				

Contd...

Contd...

Sl No	Name of the procedure	Date of demo in lab	Supervisor's signature	Date of clinical return demonstration	Clinical Supervisor signature
	Drug indent book				
	Equipment and supplies register				
	Condemnation of equipment register				
	Transfer-in and transfer-out record				
	Referral register				
	Doctors rounds, Nurses round book				
	Discharge register				
	Death register				
	Prepares reports				
	Census				
	Birth				
	Shift wise reports				
	Morbidity register				
	Recording of carried out procedures				
	Uses standardized abbreviations in charting				
	Minimizes legal liability by effective record keeping				
8	**Adopts nursing process based on nursing theories and nursing models and writes the nursing care Plan based on the needs of client**				
9	**Meeting the basic needs of a client**				
a	Utilization of comfort devices				
	Extra pillows				
	Cotton rings				
	Trochanter rolls				
	Hand rolls				
	Water bags				
	Air cushions				
	Foot rest				
	Bed cradle				
	Back rest				
	Cardiac table				
	Sand bags				

Contd...

Contd...

Sl No	Name of the procedure	Date of demo in lab	Supervisor's signature	Date of clinical return demonstration	Clinical Supervisor signature
b	Changing of positions				
	Dorsal position/supine position				
	Dorsal elevated/semirecumbent position				
	Prone position				
	Lateral/side lying position				
	Fowler's position				
	Cardiac position				
c	Positions used for physical examination				
	Supine position				
	Dorsal recumbent				
	Erect position				
	Sim's lateral or left lateral prone position				
	Lithotomy position				
	Knee-chest position				
	Trendelenburg position				
d	Activity and exercises				
	Maintenance of body mechanics				
	Maintaining body alignment, posture of the client				
	Assisting the client in ambulation				
	Assisting the client in doing active and passive exercises				
	Assisting the client in doing deep breathing and coughing exercises				
	Transferring the client from bed to wheel chair and back, trolleys				
	Bed to stretcher				
	Wheel chair to toilet seat and back				
	Using crutches				
	Using walker				
	Using wheel chair				
	Using prosthetic/orthotic devices				

Contd...

Contd...

Sl No	Name of the procedure	Date of demo in lab	Supervisor's signature	Date of clinical return demonstration	Clinical Supervisor signature
10	**Providing safe environment**				
	Maintains healthy atmosphere in the ward				
	Safe disposal of biomedical waste products				
	Uses barrier nursing technique by wearing masks, aprons, gloves				
	Adopts infection control techniques in clinical settings				
	Collection of specimens, sending for investigations and collecting reports				
11	**Health assessment**				
a	Vital signs				
	Checking and recording of vital signs				
	Temperature				
	Oral				
	Rectal				
	Axillary				
	Pulse rate at different sites				
	Respiratory pattern				
	Blood pressure in different positions				
	Level of consciousness				
12	**Assisting diagnostic measures and specific therapeutic measures**				
	Lumbar puncture				
	Venous puncture				
	Thoracentesis				
	Paracentesis				
	Duodenal and gastric suctioning				
	Gastric analysis				
	Gastric gavage and lavage				
	Electrocardiogram				
13	**Homeokinesis and Human needs**				
a	Meeting hygienic needs of the client				
	Special mouth care				
	Bed bath				

Contd...

Contd...

Sl No	Name of the procedure	Date of demo in lab	Supervisor's signature	Date of clinical return demonstration	Clinical Supervisor signature
	Back care/care related pressure points				
	Morning and Evening care (AM care and PM care)				
	Assist in bathroom bath				
	Pediculosis treatment				
	Shampooing (hair wash) for bed ridden patients				
	Hair combing				
	Offering and removal of bed pan and Urinal				
	Perineal care				
	Nail care				
	Care of hands and feet				
	Carrying out health education activities				
b	Meeting nutritional needs of clients				
	Planning and serving the therapeutic diet				
	Feeding helpless clients				
	Insertion and removal of ryles tube				
	Nasogastric tube feedings				
	Maintenance of intake and output chart				
c	Meeting elimination needs of the client				
	Catheterization				
	Care of the client with catheterization				
	Passing of flatus tube				
	Condom drainage				
	Insertion of rectal suppositories				
	Administration of soap and water enema				
	Retention enema				
	Carry out siphonage procedure				
	Colonic irrigation				
	One tube method				
	Two tube method				
	Gastric lavage				
d	Meeting the spiritual needs of the client				

Contd...

Contd...

Sl No	Name of the procedure	Date of demo in lab	Supervisor's signature	Date of clinical return demonstration	Clinical Supervisor signature
e	Measures to ensure rest and sleep among the clients				
f	Utilizes advance directives				
g	Maintains medicolegal cases and its documentation				
14	**Nursing responsibilities in therapy**				
a	Measures to relieve hyperpyrexia				
	Cold applications				
	Advising more fluids, cold drinks				
	Cold compress				
	Ice cap				
	Tepid sponging				
	Cold sponging				
b	Hot applications				
	Hot water bag				
	Medical fomentation				
	Hot packs/pads				
	Arm soak and foot soak				
	Sitz bath				
	Steam inhalation				
	Nebulization				
15	**Introduction to pharmacological therapy**				
	Calculation and preparation of drugs and solutions				
	Administration of drugs				
	Oral				
	Parenteral				
	Intramuscular injection				
	Intradermal injection				
	Subcutaneous injection				
	Hypodermic injection				
	Topical application				
	Instillation of drops in eye, ear, nose				
	Assist in infusions				
	Intravenous infusion				

Contd...

Contd...

Sl No	Name of the procedure	Date of demo in lab	Supervisor's signature	Date of clinical return demonstration	Clinical Supervisor signature
	Blood transfusion				
	Insertion of rectal suppositories				
	Inhalations				
	Steam				
	Oral				
	Prepares solution from pure to weaker solutions				
16	**Equipment and supplies**				
	Follows general principles of cleaning				
	Care of needles and syringes				
	Care of rubber goods				
	Care of patient unit				
	Care of linen				
	Care of furniture				
	Care of enamel goods				
	Stainless steel goods				
	Glassware				
	Sharp instruments				
	Maintains inventory register (equipment and linen)				
	Assists in CSSD activities for disinfection and sterilization of articles by physical methods				
	Boiling				
	Autoclaving				
	Hot air oven				
	Chemical disinfection				
	Care of equipment after-care				
17	**Care of the client with** Unconsciousness				
	Decubitus ulcer				
	Insomnia				
	Retention of urine				
	Pyrexia				

Contd...

Contd...

Sl No	Name of the procedure	Date of demo in lab	Supervisor's signature	Date of clinical return demonstration	Clinical Supervisor signature
18	**Techniques used in operation theaters**				
	Disinfection and carbolization of OT				
	Barrier nursing technique				
	Handwashing				
	Surgical scrubbing				
	Gowning				
	Gloving				
	Setting up of sterile trolleys/myostand for different surgeries				
	Assisting in autoclaving and sterilizing the OT equipment				
	Indenting and keeping ready items from CSSD				
	Preparation of different trays and packages for varied surgeries				
	Major				
	Minor				
	Storage and care of supplies and equipment for varied procedures				
	Setting up of anesthesia trolley				
	Setting up of emergency trolley				
	Care of the client in preoperative period				
	Preparation of checklist				
	Consent				
	Surgical attire				
	Medications				
	Checking and recording vital signs and weight				
	Enema (if indicated)				
	NBM				
	Psychological preparation				
	Collection of reports of investigations				
	Assisting in positioning of the client for				
	Anesthesia				
	Surgery				
	Care of the client in intraoperative period				

Contd...

Contd...

Sl No	Name of the procedure	Date of demo in lab	Supervisor's signature	Date of clinical return demonstration	Clinical Supervisor signature
	Assisting in endotracheal intubation				
	Care of the client before, during and after anesthesia				
	Assisting in tracheostomy care (if needed)				
	Assisting in pulse oximeter monitoring				
	Monitoring cardiac functioning				
	Assisting in defibrillation (if necessary)				
	Care of the client in postoperative period				
	Setting up of immediate recovery room				
	Care of the client on ventilator				
	Checking and recording of vital signs and level of consciousness				
	Suctioning				
	Oropharyngeal				
	Endotracheal				
	Oxygen administration				
	Mask				
	Oxyhood				
	Tent				
	Nasal catheter				
	Observation of oxygen toxicity				
	Care of drainage tube				
	Care of catheter				
	Meeting the needs of the client Nutritional				
	Hygienic				
	Assess the stages of wound healing				
	Assist in surgical dressing/wound dressing				
	Suture removal				
19	**Care of dying clients, care of the body after death**				
	Adopts measures to cope up with loss, grieving, death				
	Care of equipment and unit after death of a client				

Contd...

Contd...

Sl No	Name of the procedure	Date of demo in lab	Supervisor's signature	Date of clinical return demonstration	Clinical Supervisor signature
20	**Discharge procedure**				
	Intimation of follow-up care activities				
	Discharging advices				
	Assisting in rehabilitation activities				
	Recording of transfer-out cases				
21	**First aid in emergency**				
	Preparation of first aid kit				
	Cardiopulmonary resuscitation technique				
	Bandaging				
	Simple spiral				
	Reverse spiral				
	Figure of eight				
	Spica				
	Capeline, T-bandage				
	Uses Triangular bandages				
	Belts				
	Binders				
	Giving first aid for poisoning				
	Epistaxis				
	Removal of foreign bodies in eye, nose and throat				
	Providing first aid for during fracture				

Nursing Care Plans

Sl No	Care plan	Date of submission	Signature of Clinical Supervisor
1			
2			
3			
4			
5			

Ward Teaching Classes

Sl No	Topic	Date of submission	Signature of Clinical Supervisor
1			
2			
3			
4			
5			

Health Education Activities

Sl No	Topic	AV aids used	Place of presentation	Focus group	Date of presentation	Signature of Clinical Supervisor
1						
2						
3						
4						
5						

Signature of the Class Coordinator
Date:

Signature of the Principal
Date:

NUTRITION

Sl No	Name of the procedure	Date of demo in lab	Clinical Supervisor's signature
1	**Participation in nutritional survey**		
2	**Nutritional assessment/ anthropometric measurement**		
	Checking of height		
	Weight		
	Mid-arm circumference		
	Head circumference		
	Chest circumference		
3	**Selection of nutrients and planning of menu**		
4	**Preservation and storage of food**		
5	**Plans menu for focus groups by calculating RDA according to age and activity**		
6	**Preparation of balanced diet**		
	Weaning diet		
	Family diet		
7	**Therapeutic diets**		
	High-protein diet		
	High caloric diet		
	Salt restricted diet		
	Low-fat diet		
	Low-carbohydrate diet		
	Fiber diet		
8	**Preparation of recipies**		
a	Liquids/fluid diet		
	Tea/coffee		
	Fruit juice		
	Barley water		
	Lentil soup		
	Lime juice		
	Egg flip		
	Lassi		
	Dhal soup		
	Vegetable soup		
	Meat soup		
	Bone soup		

Contd...

Contd...

Sl No	Name of the procedure	Date of demo in lab	Clinical Supervisor's signature
b	Milk soup		
	Butter milk		
	Sago congee		
	Arrowroot congee		
	Orange juice		
	Tomato juice/soup		
	Grape juice		
	Light diet		
	Toast		
	Porridge		
	Salads		
	Jelly		
	Arrowroot		
	Boiled egg		
	Steamed fish		
	Omelette		
	Poached egg		
	Gruel		
	Kanji		
	Custards		
c	Vegetable preparation		
	Green leafy vegetables parota		
	Vegetable salad		
	Pachidies		
	Boiled mixed vegetable		
d	Carbohydrates		
	Rice kheer		
	Khichdi		
	Rava porridge		
	Rava upma		
	Phulka—jowar or wheat		
	Banana milk shake		
e	Proteins		
	Sprouted grams		
	Milk and egg preparations		
	Ground nut milk shake		
	Soft boiled eggs		

Contd...

Contd...

Sl No	Name of the procedure	Date of demo in lab	Clinical Supervisor's signature
	Custard		
	Steamed fish		
	Steamed meat		
	Meat curry		
	Dhal preparations		
	Vada		
f	Fats		
	Spinach bhaji		
	Wheat parota		
	Vegetable cutlet		
	Fried fish		
	Butter milk with fat		
	Pooris		
	Skimmed milk		
	Custard egg		
	Scrambled egg		
9	Methods of cooking		
	Boiling		
	Baking		
	Steaming		
	Steam under pressure		
	Frying		
	Grilling/broiling		
	Simmering		
	Roasting		
	Stewing		
10	**Feeding helpless clients**		
11	**Participated in** Community nutrition programs		
	Awareness campaigns		
	Preservation of food values		
	Nutrition research activities		
	Nutritional rehabilitation activities		

Nutrition-oriented Observational Visits

Sl No	Place of visit	Date of demo in lab	Signature of Supervisor
1	Food preservation and storage centers		
2	Food fortification center		
3	Nutritional rehabilitation home		
4	Pantries (dietary units) in hospital		
5	Food sanitation units		
6	Slaughter house		
7	Municipal market		

Signature of the Class Coordinator
Date:

Signature of the Principal
Date:

Practical Examination—I Year

Nursing Foundations

Signature of

Internal Examiner Date:

External Examiner Date:

Supplementary Examination

Signature of

Internal Examiner Date:

External Examiner Date:

II Year—Hours of Instruction

Name of the Student ....
Reg. No. ....

Total Hours: 1480

Sl No	Subjects	Theory (in hours) (Class room and Lab)	Practical/Clinical Hours	In Hours	Name of the Subject Teacher
1	Sociology	60	–	–	
2	Pharmacology	45	–	–	
3	Pathology	30	–	–	
4	Genetics	15	–	–	
5	Medical-Surgical Nursing—I (Adult including Geriatrics)	210	720	–	
6	Community Health Nursing—I	90	135	–	
7	Communication and Educational Technology	60 + 30	–	–	
8	Library Work/Self-study	–	–	50	
9	Co-curricular Activities	–	–	35	
	Total Hours	**540**	**855**	**85**	

Attendance of the Student (%) :
Theory :
Practical :
Character and Conduct :
Extra-Curricular Activities :
Co-Curricular Activities :

Signature of the Class Coordinator
Date:

Signature of the Principal
Date:

II Year—Scheme of Examination

Name of the Student ....
Reg. No. ....

Month and Year of Passing:

Sl No	Subjects	Duration of Exam in Hours		IA Marks				Marks in University Exam				Total Marks		Month and Year of Passing
				Theory		Practical		Theory		Practical				
		Theory	Practical	Max marks	Marks obtained	Max marks	Marks obtained	Max marks	Marks obtained	Max marks	Marks obtained	Total marks	Total marks obtained	
1	Sociology	3	–	25		–	–	75		-	-	100		
2	Medical -Surgical Nursing—1	3	–	25		100		75		100		T: 100 P: 200 Total: 300	T: P: Total:	
3	Pharmacology Pathology Genetics	3	–	25		–	–	75		–	–	100		
4	Community Health Nursing—I	3	–	25		–	–	75		–	–	100		
5	Communication and Education Technology	3	–	25		–	–	75		–	–	100		

- Distinction – 75% and above; I Division – 60% to 74%; II Division – 50% to 59%, Pass – 50% (Theory – 50%, Practical/Orals/Viva put together – 50%)
- 5 attempts is permitted to pass each subject; If the student failed in more than 2 subjects he/she will be detained in the same class; If 1 or 2 subjects failed, the candidate will be promoted to the next class.

Signature of the Class Coordinator
Date:

Signature of the Principal
Date:

MEDICAL-SURGICAL NURSING—I (ADULT INCLUDING GERIATRICS)

Sl No	Name of the procedure	Date of demo in lab	Supervisor's signature	Date of clinical return demonstration	Clinical Supervisor signature
1	**Clinical experience in medical wards**				
	Adopts nursing process based on nursing theories and nursing models in provision of comprehensive nursing care				
	Assessment of the patients				
	Systematically collects history of the client				
	Performs physical examination (general and specific)				
	Differentiates normal and alterations and deviations				
	Follows standard safety measures by adopting medical and surgical aseptic techniques, while providing care to the client				
	Administers medication as per prescription by following 6 'R' principle				
	Documents the administered medications				
	Prepares drug book				
	Administers intravenous infusion				
	Assists blood transfusion				
	Identification of blood donors				
	Care of blood donors				
	Counseling of blood donors				
	Maintains intake and output chart				
	Provides oxygen therapy as per the order				
	Performs chest physiotherapy				
	Provides nebulization				
	Assists in common diagnostic procedures				
	Collects the specimens and sent to the lab along with requisition				
	Collects the reports from the lab and document the findings in clinical record				
	Performs throat suctioning as per the order/ when it is needed				
	Maintains elimination				
	Performs catheterization				

Contd...

Contd...

Sl No	Name of the procedure	Date of demo in lab	Supervisor's signature	Date of clinical return demonstration	Clinical Supervisor signature
	Care of the client during catheterization				
	Administers enema as per the order				
	Counsel and teach the clients and their families about care of the clients in specific diseases				
2	**Surgical clinical experience**				
a	**Operation theaters**				
	Participates in infection control practices in OT				
	Performs disinfection, carbolization and fumigation of OT				
	Follows standard safety measures by following surgical aseptic principles				
	Adopts barrier nursing technique				
	Surgical scrubbing				
	Gowning				
	Gloving				
	Assisting in autoclaving and sterilizing the OT equipment				
	Identifies the instruments and suturing materials for common operations				
	Indenting and keeping ready items from CSSD				
	Setting up of sterile trolleys/myostand for different surgeries				
	Preparation of different trays and packages for varied surgeries, preparing OT table for varied surgeries				
	Assisting in major and minor surgeries				
	Assists in handling of specimens, sending to the lab along with requisition				
	Storage and care of supplies and equipment for varied procedures				
	Setting up of anesthesia trolley				
	Setting up of emergency trolley				
	Disposes waste as per guidelines				
b	**Care of the client in preoperative period**				
	Maintains checklist				
	Checking and recording vital signs and weight				
	Enema (if indicated)				

Contd...

Contd...

Sl No	Name of the procedure	Date of demo in lab	Supervisor's signature	Date of clinical return demonstration	Clinical Supervisor signature
	NBM				
	Psychological preparation (education and counseling)				
	Collection of reports of investigations				
	Assisting in positioning of the client for – Anesthesia				
	– Surgery				
c	**Care of the client in intraoperative period**				
	Positioning and monitoring of patients				
	Assisting in endotracheal intubation				
	Care of the client before, during and after anesthesia				
	Assisting in tracheostomy care (if needed)				
	Assisting in pulse oximeter monitoring				
	Monitoring cardiac functioning				
	Assisting in defibrillation (if necessary)				
d	**Care of the client in postoperative period**				
	Setting up of immediate recovery room				
	Provides care of the client on ventilator				
	Monitors level of consciousness and vital signs				
	Maintains Glasgow Coma Scale chart if needed				
	Performs suctioning as indicated				
	Oropharyngeal				
	Endotracheal				
	Administers oxygen				
	Mask				
	Oxyhood				
	Tent				
	Nasal catheter				
	Observes oxygen toxicity signs and symptoms				
	Provides care of drainage tube				

Contd...

Contd...

Sl No	Name of the procedure	Date of demo in lab	Supervisor's signature	Date of clinical return demonstration	Clinical Supervisor signature
	Provides care of catheter				
	Meeting the needs of the client – Nutritional				
	– Hygienic				
	Provides wound care and drainages-surgical dressing/wound dressing				
	Removes sutures				
	Assists in ambulation and exercises				
	Aspirates nasogastric tube				
	Practices universal precautions in providing care to the client in post operative period				
3	**Care of the client with cardiac disorders**				
	Monitor – Vital signs				
	– Heart sounds				
	– Breath sounds				
	Assist the client in investigative procedures				
	– Stress test				
	– Echocardiography				
	– ECG monitoring and interpretation				
	– Arterial blood gas estimation				
	– Chest X-ray and fluoroscopy				
	– Telemetry				
	– Treadmill exercise				
	– Radionuclide imaging				
	– CT scan				
	– MRI				
	– Cardiac catheterization				
	Angiography				
	Aortography				
	Arteriography				
	– Defibrillation				
	– Pulse oximetry				

Contd...

Contd...

Sl No	Name of the procedure	Date of demo in lab	Supervisor's signature	Date of clinical return demonstration	Clinical Supervisor signature
	Collection of blood for assessing cardiac enzymes				
	Pre and postoperative preparation of the client undergoing cardiac surgery				
4	**Care of the client with Skin Conditions and Communicable Diseases**				
	Assesses the clients with skin disorders				
	Assists in diagnostic and therapeutic procedures				
	Administers topical medications				
	Follows standard safety measures				
	Practices medical and surgical aseptic precautions				
	Uses personal protective equipment (PPE)				
	Provides nursing care to the clients with communicable diseases				
	Counsels HIV positive patients				
	Educates client, families and community prevention of infectious diseases				
5	**Musculoskeletal functioning**				
	Assess Posture				
	Gait				
	Reflexes				
	Bone integrity				
	Joint function				
	Muscle strength and size				
	Assisting in Imaging procedures				
	X-ray studies				
	CT scan				
	MRI				
	Arthrography				
	Bone densitometry				
	Nuclear studies				
	Endoscopy/arthroscopy				

Contd...

Contd...

Sl No	Name of the procedure	Date of demo in lab	Supervisor's signature	Date of clinical return demonstration	Clinical Supervisor signature
	Bone biopsy				
	Bone marrow aspiration				
	Estimation of serum calcium levels				
	Care of the client with Plaster of Paris/cast				
	Traction (Skin/Skeletal)				
	Stump				
	Assists in removal of cast				
	Applies skin traction, Buck's extension traction				
	Assists in application and removal of prosthesis				
	Assist the client to perform Range of motion exercises (ROM)				
	Utilizes crutch maneuvering technique				
	Assists in ADL				
	Assists in ambulation				
	Teach and counsel patients and familes in care of the clients with musuloskeletal disorders				
	Assisting in application of Splints				
	Restraints				
	Spicas				
	Bandages				
	Braces				
	Dressings				
	Assisting the client in maintenance of body alignment				
	Care of the client with fracture and other musculo-skeletal disorders				
	Care of the client with orthopedic surgeries				
	Assisting the client in performing exercises Active				
	Passive				
	Muscle strengthening				
	Assisting the client in maintaining rehabilitation activities				

Contd...

Contd...

Sl No	Name of the procedure	Date of demo in lab	Supervisor's signature	Date of clinical return demonstration	Clinical Supervisor signature
	Assist the client in crutch walking				
	Conducting health education activities regarding diet, care of cast, traction				
6	**Therapeutic diet**				
	Prepares and administers therapeutic diets				
	Implements doctor's orders in feeding the client				
	Fluid diet				
	Light diet				
	Bland diet				
	Low-fat diet				
	Salt restricted diet/low-salt diet				
	High-protein diet				
	Fluid restricted diet				
	High caloric diet				
	Fiber diet				
	Low-protein diet				
	Low-carbohydrate diet/diabetic diet				

Nursing Care Plans

Sl No	Care plan	Date of presentation	Signature of Clinical Supervisor
1			
2			
3			
4			
5			

Ward Teaching Classes

Sl No	Topic	Date of presentation	Signature of Clinical Supervisor
1			
2			
3			
4			
5			

Health Education Activities

Sl No	Topic	AV aids used	Focus group	Date of presentation	Signature of Clinical Supervisor
1					
2					
3					
4					
5					

Operation Theater Experience

Major Surgeries

Sl No	Date	Name of surgery	Assisted	Witnessed	Signature of Clinical Supervisor
1					
2					
3					
4					
5					

Minor Surgeries

Sl No	Date	Name of surgery	Assisted	Witnessed	Signature of Clinical Supervisor
1					
2					
3					
4					
5					

Signature of the Class Coordinator
Date:

Signature of the Principal
Date:

COMMUNITY HEALTH NURSING—I

Sl No	Name of the procedure	Date of demo in lab	Supervisor's signature	Date of return demonstration in lab	Clinical Supervisor's signature
1	**Mapping of the field area**				
2	**Assists in survey activities**				
	Domiciliary/household				
	Sanitary				
	Nutritional				
	Epidemiological (morbidity and mortality)				
	Communicable diseases				
	Non-communicable diseases				
	Focus group (age and sex wise)				
	Antenatal				
	Postnatal				
	Eligible couple				
3	**Community assessment**				
4	**Bag technique**				
5	**Performs home visiting**				
6	**Uses techniques of interpersonal relationship, while conducting interview within the family and community**				
7	**Health assessment of an individual in family**				
8	**Identifies health determinants of community**				
9	**Improvises equipments in home**				
10	**Monitors and records vital signs**				
11	**Implementation of community health Nursing Process**				
12	**Vital statistics**				
	Registration of Births				
	Deaths				
	Morbidity pattern				
	Age wise population				
	Sex wise population				
	Educate the community about Population education				
	Adverse effects of early age at marriage				

Contd...

Contd...

Sl No	Name of the procedure	Date of demo in lab	Supervisor's signature	Date of return demonstration in lab	Clinical Supervisor's signature
	Participate in population surveys				
	Educates adverse effects of population explosion				
13	**Family welfare services**				
	Motivating the eligible couple for adoption of family planning methods based on family size				
	Temporary FP Methods Oral pills				
	Copper T				
	Condom				
	Assisting in Copper T insertion				
	Medical Termination of Pregnancy				
	Assisting for adoption of permanent FP methods				
	Tubectomy				
	Vasectomy				
	Mini lap/laparoscopy				
	Advice on sterility				
	Investigative procedures				
	Management of sterility				
14	**Epidemiology**				
	Collects history				
	Assists in epidemiological investigations				
	Performs physical examination				
	Collects specimens like sputum, blood smears and send to the laboratory				
	Performs simple lab tests at center				
	– Blood for hemoglobin, sugar				
	– Urine for abnormal constituents like albumin, sugar				
	Actively participates in immunization activities				
	Administers vaccines				
	Maintains cold chain system				
	Utilizes barrier nursing technique				

Contd...

Contd...

Sl No	Name of the procedure	Date of demo in lab	Supervisor's signature	Date of return demonstration in lab	Clinical Supervisor's signature
	Counsel and teaches individual, family and community				
	Assists in implementation of national programs activities				
	Educates the community about The prevention and control of communicable diseases				
	Hygiene				
	Self-health monitoring				
	Seeking health services				
	Adopts healthy lifestyle				
	Health promotion measures				
	Care of the client with communicable diseases				
	Domiciliary care of TB and leprosy client				
	Motivates the client for follow-up activity for continuity of care				
	Performs scabies treatment				
	Pediculosis treatment				
15	**Meeting the specific health needs of the clients within the family**				
	– Physical needs				
	– Hygienic needs				
	– Nutritional needs				
	– Elimination needs				
	– Psychological needs				
	– Spiritual needs				
16	**Follows standards of community health nursing practice**				
17	**Treating minor ailments**				
18	**Implementation of prescribed treatments in home**				
19	**Administration of medications**				
	Oral				
	Parenteral				
	Intramuscular				
	Subcutaneous				
	Hypodermic				

Contd...

Contd...

Sl No	Name of the procedure	Date of demo in lab	Supervisor's signature	Date of return demonstration in lab	Clinical Supervisor's signature
	Intradermal				
	Assisting in intravenous infusions				
	Instillation of drugs				
	Eye				
	Ear				
	Nose				
	Eye irrigation				
	Ear irrigation				

Observational Visits

Sl No	Place of visit	Date of visit	Clinical Supervisor signature
1	FPAI		
2	Statistics departments to observe registration of vital events		
3	Epidemiology centers		
4	Isolation units		
5	TB centers		
6	Leprosy centers		
7	STD clinics		
8	Counseling centers		
9	Community health centers		
10	PHC (urban and rural)		
11	Subcenter		
12	Postpartum units		
13	Family welfare clinic		

Family Study/Family Profiles

Sl No	Family study	Date of presentation	Clinical Supervisor signature
1			
2			
3			

Family Care Plans

Sl No	Family care plan	Date of submission	Clinical Supervisor signature
1			
2			
3			

Health Education Activities

Sl No	Topic	Type of AV aids used	Place of presentation	Focus group	Date of presentation	Clinical signature of Supervisor
1						
2						
3						
4						
5						

Signature of the Class Coordinator
Date:

Signature of the Principal
Date:

Practical Examination—II Year

Medical-Surgical Nursing (Adult and Geriatric Nursing) - I

Signature of

Internal Examiner Date:

External Examiner Date:

Supplementary Examination

Signature of

Internal Examiner Date:

External Examiner Date:

III Year—Hours of Instruction

Name of the Student ....
Reg. No. ....

Total Hours: 1480

Sl No	Subjects	Theory (in hours) (Class room and Lab)	Practical/ Clinical Hours	In Hours	Name of the Subject Teacher
1	Medical-Surgical Nursing—II (Adult and Geriatrics)	150	270	–	
2	Child Health Nursing	100	270	–	
3	Mental Health Nursing	100	270	–	
4	Midwifery and Obstetrical Nursing—I	40	180	–	
5	Library Work/Self-study	–	–	50	
6	Co-curricular Activities	–	–	50	
	Total Hours	**390**	**990**	**100**	

Attendance of the Student (%) :
Theory :
Practical :
Character and Conduct :
Extra-curricular Activities :
Co-curricular Activities :

Signature of the Class Coordinator
Date:

Signature of the Principal
Date:

III Year—Scheme of Examination

Name of the Student ....

Reg. No. ....

Month and Year of Passing:

Sl No	Subjects	Duration of Exam in Hours		IA Marks				Marks in University Exam				Total Marks		Month and Year of Passing
				Theory		Practical		Theory		Practical				
		Theory	Practical	Max marks	Marks obtained	Max marks	Marks obtained	Max marks	Marks obtained	Max marks	Marks obtained	Total marks	Total marks obtained	
1	Medical-Surgical Nursing—II	3	3	25		50		75		50		T: 100 P: 100 Total: 200	T: P: Total:	
2	Child Health Nursing	3	3	25		50		75		50		T: 100 P: 100 Total: 200	T: P: Total:	
3	Mental Health Nursing	3	3	25		50		75		50		T: 100 P: 100 Total: 200	T: P: Total:	

- Distinction – 75% and above; I Division 60% to 74%, II Division – 50% to 59%, Pass – 50% (Theory – 50%, Practical/Orals/Viva put together – 50%)
- 5 attempts is permitted to pass each subject; If the student failed in more than 2 subjects he/she will be detained in the same class; If 1 or 2 subjects failed, the candidate will be promoted to the next class.

Signature of the Class Coordinator
Date:

Signature of the Principal
Date:

MIDWIFERY AND OBSTETRICAL NURSING—I

Sl No	Name of the procedure	Date of demo in lab	Supervisor's signature	Date of clinical return demonstration	Clinical Supervisor signature
1	**Fulfills the responsibility of a midwife**				
2	**Assists the woman in maternity cycle**				
3	**Educates the female adolescents about menstrual hygiene**				
4	**Setting up of the MCH and antenatal and family planning clinics**				
5	**Antenatal care**				
	Assessment of antenatal mother				
	Observation of physiological changes and clinical manifestations in pregnancy				
	Diagnoses pregnancy				
	History taking				
	Calculates expected date of delivery (EDD)				
	Assists in routine physical examination				
	Assists in investigations and ultrasonography				
	Performs abdominal examination				
	Estimates gestational age				
	Measures fundal height				
	Inspection				
	Skin changes				
	Palpation				
	Lateral				
	Fundal				
	Pelvic				
	Assess and records fetal heart sounds				
	Checking and recording of Height				
	Weight				
	Vital signs				
	Provides antenatal care/prenatal advice				
	Demonstrates antenatal exercises				
	Counseling of family members for accepting pregnancy and assist in care of antenatal mother and family adaptation				

Contd...

Contd...

Sl No	Name of the procedure	Date of demo in lab	Supervisor's signature	Date of clinical return demonstration	Clinical Supervisor signature
	Preparation of family members for Institutional delivery				
	Availability of health services and birth setting choice				
	Identification of high-risk antenatal mothers and referring them to institution				
	Guiding for adjustment to pregnancy by unwed mothers, single parent, teenage pregnancy, sexual violence				
	Care of pregnant woman with minor disorders				
6	**Normal child birth**				
	Assist in preparation of Labor unit				
	Newborn resuscitation unit				
	Admits antenatal mother to labor room				
	Assessment and monitoring of mother and fetus				
	Observe and record physiological changes and stages of labor				
	Perineal preparation of mother for labor				
	Conducts vaginal examination				
	Monitoring and recording of Uterine contractions and relaxation chart (Partograph)				
	Fetal heart sounds				
	Cervical effacement, dilatations and fetal descent				
	Signs/symptoms of labor				
	Educating the mother about Pain management				
	Breathing and relaxation exercises				
	Informal biofeedback technique				
	Psychological reassurance				
	Administration of soap and water enema				
	Maintains labor progress chart				
	Assist in Elimination activities				

Contd...

Contd...

Sl No	Name of the procedure	Date of demo in lab	Supervisor's signature	Date of clinical return demonstration	Clinical Supervisor signature
	Ambulation and positioning				
	Investigations and collecting its reports				
	Supportive measures				
	Assists in induction of labor				
	Conducts normal delivery				
	Prevents perineal tear				
	Assists in episiotomy and suturing				
	Able to perform episiotomy and suturing under clinical supervision				
	Provides perineal care				
	Adopts technique of placental expulsion				
	Monitors maternal condition				
	Observes the placenta and its membranes and records blood loss				
	Documents child birth in birth register				
	Assists in cesarian operations, MTP and other obstetrical surgical procedures				
	Provides nursing care for the women, who are undergoing obstetrical operations and procedures				
7	**Newborn care**				
	Receives newborn in sterile tray				
	Records APGAR score of newborn				
	Assessment of newborn				
	Assist in physiological adjustment of newborn				
	Provides neonatal resuscitation (if needed)				
	Provides immediate newborn care				
	Provides care to the umbilical cord				
	Assess the reflexes of newborn				
	Meets the needs of newborn				
	Provides care for high-risk newborn				
	Low birth weight babies				
	Infections				

Contd...

Contd...

Sl No	Name of the procedure	Date of demo in lab	Supervisor's signature	Date of clinical return demonstration	Clinical Supervisor signature
	Asphyxia				
	Birth injuries				
	Respiratory problems				
	Hemolytic disorders				
	Malformations				
	Care of the neonate in Phototherapy unit				
	Radiant warmer				
	Ventilator				
	Incubator				
	Performs assistance in neonatal intensive care units				
	Adopts infection control in neonatal intensive care units				
	Maintains records and reports				
8	**Conducts normal home delivery**				
	Care of newborn				
	Educate the mother about the importance of 'kangaroo mother care'				
9	**Postpartum care**				
	Assess and records changes in postnatal period of a mother Involution of uterus				
	Uterine contractions				
	After pains				
	Lochia changes				
	Changes in cervix				
	Lactation				
	Provides postnatal care				
	Provides perineal care				
	Assist the mother for – Newborn care				
	– Postnatal exercises				
	– Care of the breast				
	Registers birth				

Contd...

Contd...

Sl No	Name of the procedure	Date of demo in lab	Supervisor's signature	Date of clinical return demonstration	Clinical Supervisor signature
	Assists the mother for promotion of comfort				
	– Rest				
	– Ambulation and exercise				
	– High-protein, caloric and vitamin rich diet				
	– Breastfeeding				
	– Normal bowel and bladder patterns				
	– Adjusts the family members for newborn arrival				
	– Immunizes the child				
	Health education activities carried out related to customs and beliefs in relation to confinement of lactation				
	Educating mother in the preparation of weaning diet				
10	**Drugs in common use**				
	Prepares drug book				
	Maintains standing orders of midwifery				
11	**Family Planning**				
	Assists and counsels the eligible couple for family welfare services				
	Educates the eligible couple about suitable family planning methods				
	Motivates the eligible couple to adopt family planning methods				
	Utilize counseling technique to motivate the eligible couple				
	Assists in FP clinics functioning				
	Assists in IUD insertion				
	Assists in OT during vasectomy, tubectomy, Minilap operations				
	Maintains FP registers and reports				

Observational Visits

Sl No	Place of visit	Date	Signature of Clinical Supervisor
1	MCH clinic		
2	Antenatal clinic		
3	Postpartum center		
4	Family planning clinic		
5	Sterility centers		
6	FPAI		

Nursing Care Plans

Sl No	Care plan	Date of submission	Signature of Clinical Supervisor
1			
2			
3			
4			
5			

Case Presentations

Sl No	Diagnosis of case	Date of presentation	Signature of Clinical Supervisor
1			
2			
3			
4			
5			

Health Education Activities

Sl No	Topic	Type of AV aids used	Place of presentation	Focus group	Date of presentation	Clinical signature of Supervisor
1						
2						
3						
4						
5						

Essential Requirements for Registration as a Midwife

1	Antenatal examination	30
2	Conducting normal deliveries in hospital/home/health center	20
3	Vaginal examination	05
4	Episiotomy and suturing	05
5	Neonatal resuscitation	05
6	Assist in cesarean section	02
7	Assist or witness abnormal deliveries	05
8	Provide postnatal care for the mothers in hospital/home/health center	20
9	Insertion of IUD	05
10	Submits case book	

Signature of the Class Coordinator
Date:

Signature of the Principal
Date:

MEDICAL-SURGICAL NURSING (ADULT and GERIATRICS)—II

Sl No	Name of the procedure	Date of demo in lab	Supervisor's signature	Date of Clinical return demonstration	Clinical Supervisor signature
1	**Ear functioning**				
	Assists in conducting auditory function tests				
	– Finger friction test				
	– Watch test				
	– Speech test				
	– Tuning fork test				
	– Rinne test				
	– Weber test				
	– Absolute bone conduction test				
	– Schwabach test				
	– Bing test				
	– Gelle test				
	Audiometric tests				
	– Pure tone audiometry				
	– Speech audiometry				
	– Tympanometry				
	– Acoustic reflex measurement				
	– Radiological examination				
	Assists with therapeutic procedures				
	Instills ear drops				
	Performs ear irrigation				
	Sending specimen of ear discharge for culture and sensitivity				
	Collects the reports and informs to the doctor				
	Provides care of the client with ear disorders				
	Applies ear bandage				
	Assisting the client in usage of hearing aid				
	Provides first aid for foreign body in the ear				
	Rehabilitation of the hearing impaired				
	Teach the clients and families about care of the client during ear disorders				

Contd...

Contd...

Sl No	Name of the procedure	Date of demo in lab	Supervisor's signature	Date of Clinical return demonstration	Clinical Supervisor signature
2	**Nasal functioning**				
	Functional examination of nose				
	Patency of nose—spatula and cotton wool test				
	Sense of smell				
	Assisting in procedures related to nasal cavity				
	Rhinoscopy				
	Nasopharyngoscopy				
	Radiography				
	Nasal secretions for culture and sensitivity				
	CT scan				
	Biopsy				
	Assists the client for therapeutic procedures				
	Sending specimen of nasal discharge for culture and sensitivity, collects the reports and informs to the doctor				
	Instills nasal drops				
	Provides first aid in controlling epistaxis and foreign body in nose				
	Assessing tonsillar size, symmetry				
	Provides care for the client with nasal deformities				
3	**Throat functioning**				
	Assessing the lymph nodes sizes and enlargement				
	Collection of specimens for culture and sensitivity				
	Sputum				
	Throat swab				
	Assisting in Bronchoscopy				
	Indirect tracheoscopy				
	Mediastinoscopy				
	Radiography				
	CT scan				
	Esophagoscopy				
	Collects the reports and informs to the doctor				
	Performs tracheostomy care				

Contd...

Contd...

Sl No	Name of the procedure	Date of demo in lab	Supervisor's signature	Date of Clinical return demonstration	Clinical Supervisor signature
	Teach the clients and families in taking care of the client with throat disorders				
4	**Ophthalmic functioning**				
	Assist the client in Testing of visual acuity				
	Fundoscopy				
	Regurgitation test				
	Lacrimal syringing				
	Measurement of intraocular pressure/ tonometry				
	Syringing				
	Ophthalmoscopy				
	Ophthalmometry				
	Perimetry				
	Fundus fluorescein angiography				
	Refraction tests				
	Retinoscopy				
	Refractometry				
	Gonioscopy				
	Care of the client with ophthalmic disorders				
	Assist for Cataract surgery				
	Laser trabeculoplasty				
	Other ophthalmic surgeries				
	Assist the client for usage of contact lens				
	Administration of vitamin A drops to under 3 years of age child				
	Instills eye drops				
	Performs eye irrigation procedure				
	Applies eye bandage				
	Provides care to the client with eye disorders				
	Provides first aid for removal of foreign body in the eye				
	Educates the client and family about care of the client with eye disorders				

Contd...

Contd...

Sl No	Name of the procedure	Date of demo in lab	Supervisor's signature	Date of Clinical return demonstration	Clinical Supervisor signature
	Provides care to the client in preoperative, postoperative period of eye surgeries				
5	**Neurological functioning**				
	Assess neurological functioning of the client and records findings				
	Maintains glasgow coma scale chart				
	Collects/assists in sending the specimens along with requisition to the lab and collects its reports, notifies to the doctor during rounds				
	Assists in investigative procedures – Lumbar puncture				
	– Cisternal puncture				
	– Histopathological biopsy				
	X-ray – Spine				
	– Skull				
	Cerebral angiography				
	Pneumoencephalography				
	Ventriculopuncture				
	Myelography				
	Ventriculogram				
	EEG				
	Electromyography				
	CT scan				
	MRI				
	Brain scan				
	Arteriography				
	Assists with therapeutic procedures				
	Provides care of the client with – Brain infections				
	– Spinal cord infections				
	– Brain and spinal cord tumors				
	– Head injury				
	– Paralysis				

Contd...

Contd...

Sl No	Name of the procedure	Date of demo in lab	Supervisor's signature	Date of Clinical return demonstration	Clinical Supervisor signature
	– CVA				
	– Status epilepticus				
	Provides pre- and postoperative care of the client with neurosurgeries				
	Assists the client for rehabilitation activities				
	Providing first aid during epileptic attacks				
	Provide care of the client with degenerative disorders				
	Provide care of the client with cranial nerve disorders				
	Educate the clients and their families about care of the clients with neurological disorders				
	Assists the client in rehabilitation programs				
6	**Assist in examination of a gynecological patient**				
	History taking				
	Gynecological examination				
	Breast examination				
	Abdominal examination				
	Pelvic examination				
	Clinical investigations				
	Assists with PAP smear collection				
	Assist in Colposcopy				
	X-ray				
	Ultrasonography				
	CT scan				
	MRI				
	Biopsy				
	Laparoscopy				
	Hysteroscopy				
	Salpingoscopy				
	Cystoscopy				
	Culdoscopy				

Contd...

Contd...

Sl No	Name of the procedure	Date of demo in lab	Supervisor's signature	Date of Clinical return demonstration	Clinical Supervisor signature
	Proctoscopy				
	Electronic monitoring				
	Assist the woman with gynecological problems				
7	**Burns and scalds**				
	Estimates percentage and degree of burns				
	Calculation of fluid requirement for burn cases				
	Calculates the fluid requirement and administers fluids and electrolytes				
	Maintain intake and output chart				
	Provides first aid				
	Assists in wound dressing				
	Utilizes barrier technique				
	Preparation of client for reconstructive surgery and donor area				
8	**Cancer disorders**				
	Assists in screening of the clients with common cancers				
	Assists the clients in diagnostic procedures Biopsies				
	PAP smear collection				
	Conducts breast examination				
	Bone marrow aspirations				
	Assists in carrying out the therapeutic procedures				
	Assists in varied modalities of treatment				
	Educates the client and family about uses and side effects of drugs and care of the client during chemotherapy				
	Educates the client and family about purposes and care of the client during radiotherapy				
	Assists and educates the client in pain management				
	Assists the clent in Stomal therapy				
	Hormonal therapy				
	Immuno therapy				
	Gene Therapy				

Contd...

Contd...

Sl No	Name of the procedure	Date of demo in lab	Supervisor's signature	Date of Clinical return demonstration	Clinical Supervisor signature
	Alternative therapy				
	Palliative care				
	Counsels and educates the clients and their families in care				
	Educates the client in breast self-examination				
	Teach the client and families about warning signs				
	Participates in rehabilitation programs				
9	**Critical care unit**				
	Monitors the clients in ICU.				
	Maintains flow sheet				
	Provides care of the clients on ventilators				
	Performs endotracheal suction				
	Collects specimens and sends to the lab along with requisition				
	Collects the reports and interprets ABG analysis				
	Assists with arterial puncture				
	Maintains CVP line				
	Interprets pulse oximetry results				
	Provides CPR whenever needed				
	Assists in defrillation , pacemaker implantation				
	Keeps ready emergency tray				
	Administers the drugs by infusion pump and total parentral therapy and maintains I/O chart				
	Performs chest physiotherapy				
	Performs active and passive exercises				
	Assists the client and family in dealing with grieving and bereavement				
10	**Casualty/emergency**				
	Practices triage				
	Assists in examination in investigations and their interpretations in emergency and disaster situations				
	Documents the findings and reports to the doctor				

Contd...

Contd...

Sl No	Name of the procedure	Date of demo in lab	Supervisor's signature	Date of Clinical return demonstration	Clinical Supervisor signature
	Assists in legal procedures in emergency unit				
	Manages crowd				
	Counsels the client and families in grief and bereavement				

Nursing Care Plans

Sl No	Care plan	Date of submission	Signature of Clinical Supervisor
1			
2			
3			
4			
5			

Case Presentations

Sl No	Diagnosis of case	Date of presentation	Signature of Clinical Supervisor
1			
2			
3			
4			
5			

Ward Teaching Classes

Sl No	Topic	Date of presentation	Signature of Clinical Supervisor
1			
2			
3			
4			
5			

Health Education Activities

Sl No	Topic	Type of AV aids used	Place of presentation	Focus group	Date of presentation	Clinical signature of Supervisor
1						
2						
3						
4						
5						

Operation Theater Experience

Major Surgeries

Sl No	Date	Name of surgery	Assisted	Witnessed	Signature of Clinical Supervisor
1					
2					
3					
4					
5					

Minor Surgeries

Sl No	Date	Name of surgery	Assisted	Witnessed	Signature of Clinical Supervisor
1					
2					
3					
4					
5					

Signature of the Class Coordinator
Date:

Signature of the Principal
Date:

CHILD HEALTH NURSING

Sl No	Name of the procedure	Date of demo in lab	Super-visor's signature	Date of Clinical return demonstration	Clinical Supervisor's signature
1	**Assist in setting up of pediatric OPD and pediatric wards (Medical and Surgical)**				
2	**Admits the sick child in pediatric unit**				
3	**Assess the childs' health status**				
a	Collects the child's history completely				
b	Conducts thoroughly physical examination from head to foot				
c	Anthropometric measurements				
	Checks weight of the child				
	Measures–length/height of child				
	– Head circumference				
	– Chest circumference				
	– Mid-upper arm circumference				
	Maintains growth chart (road to health chart)				
d	Assess child's development and document findings				
	Maintains the developmental screening chart				
	Physical				
	Emotional				
	Social				
	Moral				
	Spiritual				
	Language and speech				
	Intellectual				
	Sexual				
e	Family assessment				
4	**Applies nursing process in the care of children**				
5	**Monitor and records the vital signs**				
	Temperature				
	Oral				
	Auxillary				
	Rectal				
	Pulse rate				
	Respiratory pattern				
	Blood pressure				

Contd...

Contd...

Sl No	Name of the procedure	Date of demo in lab	Super-visor's signature	Date of Clinical return demonstration	Clinical Supervisor's signature
6	**Feeding of the child**				
	Assist in breastfeeding and bottle feeding				
	Supplements weaning diet				
	Planning of special diet/menu for needy children				
	Feeds the child through nasogastric tube (if indicated)				
	Feeds the client with cleft lip and cleft palate				
	Provides gastrostomy feeding				
7	**Administers the medications as per order**				
	Oral				
	Parenteral				
	Intramuscular injection				
	Intradermal injection				
	Subcutaneous injection				
	Hypodermic injection				
	Assist in intravenous infusion				
	Assist in blood transfusion				
	Calculates the flow rates for intravenous fluid administration				
	Inserts the rectal suppositories				
	Assists in administering intrathecal injection				
	Instill the drops in eyes, nose, ear				
	Applies topical ointments				
	Provides steam inhalation and nebulization				
8	**Uses the restraints**				
9	**Collects the specimens and sending to lab and collecting reports**				
10	**Assist in performing special investigative procedures**				
	Lumbar puncture				
	Exchange transfusion				
	Painful procedures				
11	**Participates in therapeutic activities** Play therapy				
	Recreational therapy				
	Diversional therapy				
	Drug therapy				

Contd...

Contd...

Sl No	Name of the procedure	Date of demo in lab	Super-visor's signature	Date of Clinical return demonstration	Clinical Supervisor's signature
12	**Pediatric emergencies**				
	Care of the child in Incubator				
	Radiant warmer				
	Phototherapy unit				
	Provide care to the high-risk children • Hemolytic disorder				
	• Preterm baby				
	• Convulsions				
	• Newborn with asphyxia				
	• Head injury				
	• Accidents				
	• On ventilator				
	Provides cardiopulmonary resuscitation				
13	**Administers oxygen (if indicated)**				
	Oxyhood				
	Tent				
	Mask				
	Nasal catheter				
	Observe the child for oxygen toxicity				
14	**Provides preoperative care for the child**				
15	**Provides postoperative care for the child**				
16	**Provides care for the child in NICU, PICU**				
17	**Genetics**				
	Identifies the chromosomal abnormalities				
	Provides care for the child with genetic disorder				
	Does pedigree charting				
	Provides genetic counseling				
	Identifies the normal child and sick child				
18	**Newborn**				
	Assessment of newborn				
	Assists in adjustment of newborn				
	Assists in neonatal resuscitation				
	Provides immediate care for the newborn				
	– Warmth (mummification)				

Contd...

Contd...

Sl No	Name of the procedure	Date of demo in lab	Super-visor's signature	Date of Clinical return demonstration	Clinical Supervisor's signature
	– Protection				
	– Cord care				
	– Baby bath				
	– Rooming-in				
	Assesses the neonatal reflexes				
	Immunizes the newborn with zero dose vaccines				
	Identifies and provide care for high-risk neonates				
	– Low birth weight child in incubators				
	– Congenital malformations				
	Provides kangaroo mother care				
	Provides integrated management of neonatal and childhood diseases				
19	**Infant**				
	Assesses the infant growth and develoment				
	Assesses the infant's reflexes				
	Immunizes the child				
	Assists in selection of toys, stimulates infant for play activities				
	Meeting the infant needs				
	Assisting the mother in preparation of weaning diet, feeding with katori, spoon, etc.				
20	**Toddler**				
	Assesses the growth and development				
	Meeting the needs of the toddler				
	Assist the child for toilet training				
	Assist the family members in prevention of accidents				
	Stimulates the toddler for play activities				
	Immunizes the child with booster doses				
21	**Preschool child**				
	Assesses the growth and development				
	Assists in selection of toys and types of play				
	Meeting the needs of preschool child				

Contd...

Contd...

Sl No	Name of the procedure	Date of demo in lab	Super-visor's signature	Date of Clinical return demonstration	Clinical Supervisor's signature
22	**School-age child**				
	Assessment of growth and development				
	Meeting the needs of school-age child				
	Provides emotional preparation of the parents for success of their child in school				
	Provides care for the child with behavior problems				
23	**Adolescents**				
	Preparing the child for accepting secondary sexual characteristics				
	Educating adolescents about Sex education				
	Extracurricular activities				
	Menstrual hygiene				
	Meeting the needs of adolescents				
	Provides guidance and counseling services for the child with behavior problems				
24	**Play activities**				
	Assists in selection of toys for different age groups				
	Assists the child in different types of play therapeutic activities				
	Identifies the imbalances in play activities in children				
25	**Assessment of dehydration status**				
	Replacement of fluids according to the level of dehydration				
	Preparation of ORS solution and supplementation of fluids in dehydration				
	Assist in intravenous infusions				
	Maintains intake and output chart				
26	**Integumentary system**				
	Calculates percentage and degree of burns in children				
	Assess dehydration				
	Calculates the flow rate for fluid replacement				

Contd...

Contd...

Sl No	Name of the procedure	Date of demo in lab	Super-visor's signature	Date of Clinical return demonstration	Clinical Supervisor's signature
	Assists in wound dressing				
	Provides scabies treatment				
	Provide care to the client with skin disorders				
27	**Communicable diseases**				
	Participates in prevention and control of communicable diseases				
	Provides nursing care of the child with communicable diseases				
	Provides nursing care for the child with HIV/AIDS				
28	**Musculoskeletal system functioning**				
	Monitor the child gait, posture, joint movements				
	Care of the child with – Club foot				
	– Hip dysplasia				
	– Genu varum (bow knee)				
	– Genu valgum (knock knee)				
	– Arthritis and arthralgia				
29	**Gastrointestinal system**				
	Assesses the nutritional status				
	Assess the rectal examination for perianal abnormalities				
	Assess for hernial sites				
	Provides care of the child with colostomy				
	Provides care of the child with GIT disorders and nutritional disorders				
	Monitors the child for nutritional deficiency symptom				
	Provides therapeutic diet				
	Assist in supplementation of nutrients to the children by specific child welfare agencies				
	Administers vitamin A solution for the below 3 year child				
	Carryout health education activities				
	Provides care for the child with PEM and other deficiency disorders				

Contd...

Contd...

Sl No	Name of the procedure	Date of demo in lab	Super-visor's signature	Date of Clinical return demonstration	Clinical Supervisor's signature
30	**Respiratory system**				
	Observes the respiratory pattern				
	Provides care for the child with respiratory problems				
	Provides care for the child with tracheostomy				
31	**Cardiovascular system**				
	Conducts general physical examination and observes the level of comfort				
	Monitors vital signs				
	– Pulse pattern—rate, volume, rhythm, character				
	– Peripheral pulses				
	– Sleeping pulse rate				
	– Lymphadenopathy				
	– Edema				
	– Clubbing of fingers				
	– Skin changes				
	– Inflammatory signs/symptoms				
	– Heart sounds				
	– Fluid thrills				
	Provides care for the child with congenital defects				
	Provides care for the child with cardiovascular problems				
	Provides care for the child with hematological disorders				
32	**Central nervous system**				
	Conducts general physical examination and observes the appearance				
	– Level of consciousness				
	– Orientation				
	– Memory pattern				
	– Speech pattern				
	– Nature of disability				
	– Symmetry of skull				
	– Fontanels				

Contd...

Contd...

Sl No	Name of the procedure	Date of demo in lab	Super-visor's signature	Date of Clinical return demonstration	Clinical Supervisor's signature
	– Signs/symptoms of increased ICP				
	– Lymphadenopathy				
	Assess cranial nerves functioning				
	Sensorymotor functioning, reflexes				
	Coordination of movements				
	Eye movement				
	Autonomic nervous system functioning				
	Salivation				
	Lacrimation				
	Sweating				
	Provides care for the child with Meningitis				
	Encephalitis				
	Cerebral palsy				
	Hydrocephalus				
	Tumors				
33	**Endocrine system**				
	Assist in hormonal assay				
	Provides care for the child with juvenile diabetes and other hormonal disorders				
34	**Care of the child with behavioral and social problems**				
	Provides care for the child with behavioral problems				
	Provides care for the child with common psychiatric problems				
	Provides care for the child with challenged children				
	Assists to identify the social welfare agencies to provide services for challenged children				
	Assists in child guidance clinics				
35	**Provides care for the child with genitorurinary disorders**				
36	**Participates in** Immunization activities and maintaining cold chain system				
	School health services				

Contd...

Contd...

Sl No	Name of the procedure	Date of demo in lab	Super-visor's signature	Date of Clinical return demonstration	Clinical Supervisor's signature
	RCH program activities				
	CSSM program activities				
	Child health program activities				
	National Nutritional Programs				
	Child to child approach				
	Under-five children survey				
	Parental guidance clinics				
	Morbidity and mortality surveys				
	Genetic counseling				
37	**Provides nursing care for the child with health emergencies**				
38	**Provides first aid for the child with** Drowning				
	Poisoning				
	Hemorrhage				
	Foreign bodies				
	Burns and scalds				
39	**Provides care for the child in pediatric surgical unit**				
	Assist in performing bowel wash				
	Provides care of the child with ostomies				
	Provides care of the child with catheterization				
	Provide feedings by – Nasogastric tube				
	– Gastrostomy				
	– Enterostomy				
	Provides wound care				
	Assists in suture removal				
	Maintains intake and output chart				
40	**Conducts health educational activities in OPDs**				
41	**Provides nursing care for critically ill children in pediatric intensive care units**				
	Monitor and document baby condition, reports to the doctor if needed				
	Performs endotracheal suctioning				

Contd...

Contd...

Sl No	Name of the procedure	Date of demo in lab	Super-visor's signature	Date of Clinical return demonstration	Clinical Supervisor's signature
	Performs chest physiotherapy				
	Administers fluids with infusion pumps				
	Assists in total parentral nutrition				
	Provides CPR				

Observational Visits

Sl No	Place of visit	Date of visit	Clinical Supervisor signature
1	Child guidance clinic		
2	MCH clinic		
3	Under-five clinic		
4	Well baby clinic		
5	Balwadi center		
6	Anganwadi center		
7	Guidance and counseling center		
8	ICDS centers		
9	Baby-friendly hospitals		
10	Child welfare agencies		
11	Delinquent homes		
12	Handicapped homes		
13	Remand homes/certified schools		
14	Crèche		
15	Nutritional guidance clinic		
16	Nursery school		
17	Play home		

Nursing Care Plans

Sl No	Care plan	Date of submission	Signature of Clinical Supervisor
1			
2			
3			

Case Presentations

Sl No	Diagnosis of case	Date of presentation	Signature of Clinical Supervisor
1			
2			
3			
4			
5			

Ward Teaching Classes

Sl No	Topic	Date of presentation	Signature of Clinical Supervisor
1			
2			
3			
4			
5			

Health Education Activities

Sl No	Topic	AV aids used	Place of presentation	Focus group	Date of presentation	Signature of Supervisor
1						
2						
3						
4						
5						

Signature of the Class Coordinator
Date:

Signature of the Principal
Date:

MENTAL HEALTH NURSING

Sl No	Name of the procedure	Date of performance	Clinical Supervisor signature
1	**Assists in admission of the client to a psychiatric unit**		
2	**Collects complete history of the client**		
3	**Performs mental status examination**		
4	**Assists in psychometric assessment**		
5	**Performs neurological examination**		
6	**Maintains standards of mental health nursing**		
7	**Follows principles of psychiatric nursing**		
8	**Establishes therapeutic nurse-patient relationship**		
9	**Follows legal aspects in provision of mental health services**		
10	**Able to differentiate normative and abnormal behavior**		
11	**Adapts process recording**		
12	**Educates the client and family about the principles of levels of prevention**		
13	**Applies various nursing theories and nursing models in provision of care**		
14	**Informs the clients and his family members about** – The availability of mental health services		
	– Community agencies and resources for client welfare		
	– Psychiatric illnesses and treatment		
15	**Provides therapeutic environment for the client**		
16	**Observes and Assists in provision of therapeutic modalities**		
	Physical therapies		
	Care of the client before, during and after ECT		
	Abreactive therapy		
	Psychotherapy		
	Individual		
	Group		
	Behavior therapy		
	Hypnosis		
	Counseling		
	Psychoanalysis		

Contd...

Contd...

Sl No	Name of the procedure	Date of performance	Clinical Supervisor signature
	Diversional therapy		
	Family therapy		
	Care of the client in drug therapy		
	Prepares the drug chart		
	Assists in activity therapy		
	– Occupation therapy		
	– Music therapy		
	– Dance therapy		
	– Psychodrama		
	– Recreational therapy		
	– Play therapy		
	– Rehabilitation activities		
17	**Provides care for the client with** – Organic disorders		
	– Functional disorders		
	– Childhood psychiatric disorders.		
	– Psychiatric emergencies		
18	**Care of the child with psychiatric problems**		
19	**Participates in the activities related to prevention and control of mental illness**		
20	**Discharges the client from psychiatric hospital**		
	Provides follow-up services		
	Provides continuity of services at community level		
21	**Prevents potential problems of mental illness in the community**		
22	**Participates in community mental health activities**		
23	**Counsel and teach patients and family members and significant others about psychiatric illnesses**		
24	**Child guidance clinic**		
	Assess the children with various mental health problems		
	Counsel and educate children, families and significant others		

Contd...

Sl No	Name of the procedure	Date of performance	Clinical Supervisor signature
25	**Community Psychiatry**		
	Identifies the clients with various mental disorders		
	Motivates the patients for early treatment and follow-up		
	Conducts case work		
	Assists in – Follow-up clinic		
	– Mental health clinics		
	– Mental health camps		
	Counsels and educate the patient, family and community		

Observational Visits

Sl No	Place of visit	Date of visit	Signature of Clinical Supervisor
1	Psychiatry speciality units		
2	Rehabilitation centers		
3	Community mental health centers		
4	Certified schools/remand homes		
5	Old age homes		
6	Delinquent homes		
7	Halfway homes		
8	Drug de-addiction centers		
9	Home for mentally retarded		
10	Group home		
11	Foster home		
12	Day care center		
13	Sheltered workshop		
14	Industrial mental health services		
15	School mental health services		

Nursing Care Plans

Sl No	Care plan	Date of submission	Signature of Clinical Supervisor
1			
2			
3			
4			
5			

Case Presentations

Sl No	Diagnosis of case	Date of presentation	Signature of Clinical Supervisor
1			
2			
3			
4			
5			

Ward Teaching Classes

Sl No	Topic	Date of presentation	Signature of Clinical Supervisor
1			
2			
3			
4			
5			

Health Education Activities

Sl No	Topic	Type of AV aids used	Place of presentation	Focus group	Date of presentation	Signature of Clinical Supervisor
1						
2						
3						
4						
5						

List of Rehabilitation Activities Assisted/Witnessed

Sl No	Rehabilitation activities	Signature of Clinical Supervisor
1		
2		
3		
4		
5		

Signature of the Class Coordinator
Date:

Signature of the Principal
Date:

Practical Examination—III Year

1. **Midwifery and Obstetrical Nursing—I**

Signature of

Internal Examiner Date:

External Examiner Date:

Supplementary Examination

Signature of

Internal Examiner Date:

External Examiner Date:

2. **Child Health Nursing**

Signature of

Internal Examiner Date:

External Examiner Date:

Supplementary Examination

Signature of

Internal Examiner Date:

External Examiner Date:

3. **Medical-Surgical Nursing—II (Adult and Geriatrics)**

Signature of

Internal Examiner Date:

External Examiner Date:

Supplementary Examination

Signature of

Internal Examiner Date:

External Examiner Date:

4. **Mental Health Nursing**

Signature of

Internal Examiner Date:

External Examiner Date:

Supplementary Examination

Signature of

Internal Examiner Date:

External Examiner Date:

IV Year—Hours of Instruction

Name of the Student ....
Reg. No. ....

Total Hours: 600

Sl No	Subjects	Theory (in hours) (Class room and Lab)	Practical/ Clinical Hours	In Hours	Name of the Subject Teacher
1	Midwifery and Obstetrical Nursing—II	60	180	–	
2	Community Health Nursing—II	90	135	–	
3	Nursing Research and Statistics	45	*	–	
4	Management of Nursing Services and Education	60 + 30	–	–	
	Total Hours	**285**	**315**		

Project work has to be carried out during internship

Attendance of the Student (%) :
Theory :
Practical :
Character and Conduct :
Extra-curricular Activities :
Co-curricular Activities :

Signature of the Class Coordinator
Date:

Signature of the Principal
Date:

IV Year—Scheme of Examination

Name of the Student ....
Reg. No. ....

Month and Year of Passing:

Sl No	Subjects	Duration of Exam in Hours		IA Marks				Marks in University Exam				Total Marks		Month and Year of Passing
				Theory		Practical		Theory		Practical				
		Theory	Practical	Max marks	Marks obta-ined	Max marks	Marks obta-ined	Max marks	Marks obta-ined	Max marks	Marks obta-ined	Total marks	Total marks obta-ined	
1	Midwifery and Obstetrical Nursing—II	3	3	25		50		75		50		T: 100 P: 100 Total: 200	T: P: Total:	
2	Community Health Nursing—II	3	3	25		50		75		50		T: 100 P: 100 Total: 200	T: P: Total:	
3	Management of Nursing Services and Education	3	–	25		–	–	75		100		100		

- Distinction – 75% and above; I Division – 60% to 74%; II Division – 50% to 59%, Pass – 50% (Theory – 50%, Practical/Orals/Viva put together – 50%)
- 5 attempts is permitted to pass each subject; If the student failed in more than 2 subjects he/she will be detained in the same class; If 1 or 2 subjects failed, the candidate will be promoted to the next class.

Signature of the Class Coordinator
Date:

Signature of the Principal
Date:

MIDWIFERY AND OBSTETRICAL NURSING—II

Sl No	Name of the procedure	Date of demo in lab	Supervisor's signature	Date of clinical return demonstration	Clinical Supervisor signature
1	**Abnormal pregnancy and management**				
	Assists in setting-up of eclampsia unit				
	Provides care to the pregnant women with abnormal pregnancy				
	Provides care to the pregnant woman complicated by gynecological conditions				
	Provides care to the pregnant woman with AIDS				
2	**Abnormal labor and management**				
	Assists in labor cases with abnormal presentations				
	Occipitoposterior				
	Breech				
	Face				
	Shoulder				
	Provides care to the mother with multiple pregnancies and obstetric emergencies				
	Assist in prolonged pregnancy Induction of labor				
	Prolonged labor				
	Obstructed labor				
	Assists in obstetric operations Manual removal of placenta				
	Version				
	Episiotomy				
	Forceps delivery				
	Vacuum extraction				
	Cesarean operation				
	Dilation and curettage				
	MTP				
	Hysterectomy				
	Laparoscopy				
	Embryotomy				

Contd...

Contd...

Sl No	Name of the procedure	Date of demo in lab	Supervisor's signature	Date of clinical return demonstration	Clinical Supervisor signature
3	**Provides care for the women during complications of 3rd stage of labor**				
4	Provides care of women in – Precipitated labor				
	– PRM				
	– Injuries to birth canal				
	– Provides care of the child with HIV infection				
5	**Provides care of the postnatal mother with abnormal puerperium**				
6	**Gynecological Nursing**				
	Assist in examination of a gynecological patient				
	History taking				
	Gynecological examination				
	Breast examination				
	Abdominal examination				
	Pelvic examination				
	Clinical investigations				
	• PAP smear				
	• Assist in–colposcopy – X-ray				
	– Ultrasonography				
	– CT scan				
	– MRI				
	– Biopsy				
	– Laparoscopy				
	– Hysteroscopy				
	– Salpingoscopy				
	– Cystoscopy				
	– Culdoscopy				
	– Proctoscopy				
	– Electronic monitoring				
	Assist the woman with gynecological problems				

Contd...

Contd...

Sl No	Name of the procedure	Date of demo in lab	Supervisor's signature	Date of clinical return demonstration	Clinical Supervisor signature
	Assist the woman with investigative procedures and management of sterility				
	Provides care of the woman with – Menstrual disorders				
	– Ovarian cysts				
	– Uterine polyps				
	– Uterine tumors				
	– Vaginal fistulas				
	– Congenital deformities				
	Assist the woman in use of T-binders				

Nursing Care Plans

Sl No	Care plan	Date of submission	Signature of Clinical Supervisor
1			
2			
3			
4			
5			

Case Presentations

Sl No	Diagnosis of case	Date of presentation	Signature of Clinical Supervisor
1			
2			
3			
4			
5			

Health Education Activities

Sl No	Topic	Type of AV aids used	Place of presentation	Focus group	Date of presentation	Clinical signature of Supervisor
1						
2						
3						
4						
5						

Signature of the Class Coordinator
Date:

Signature of the Principal
Date:

COMMUNITY HEALTH NURSING—II

Sl No	Name of the procedure	Date of demo	Date of return demonstration	Clinical Supervisor signature
1	**Mapping of the field area**			
2	**Assists in survey activities**			
	Domiciliary/household			
	Sanitary			
	Nutritional			
	Epidemiological			
	Communicable diseases			
	Non-communicable diseases			
	Focus group (age and sex wise)			
	Antenatal			
	Postnatal			
	Eligible couple			
3	**Performs community assessment**			
4	**Identifies community profile**			
5	**Performs homevisit**			
6	**Utilizes bag technique to provide care for the people at home**			
7	**Maintains good interpersonal skills, develops rapport and gathers data by conducting focus group interview**			
8	**Conducts health assessment and diagnoses the health needs of individual, family and community**			
	Monitoring milestones of children's growth and development			
	Checking and recording vital signs			
	Breast self-examination			
	Warning signs of various diseases			
	Testing of urine for abnormal constituents like albumin and sugar			
	Seeking health services for Routine checkup			
	Counseling			
	Diagnosis, treatment and follow-up			
	Continue medical care in community for disabilities and diseases			

Contd...

Contd...

Sl No	Name of the procedure	Date of demo	Date of return demonstration	Clinical Supervisor signature
9	**Improvises equipments in home in provision of care to the needy people in home**			
10	**Meet the specific health needs of the clients within the family** – Physical needs			
	– Emotional needs			
	– Social needs			
	– Spiritual needs			
11	**Follows standards of Community Health Nursing Practice**			
12	**Treats minor ailments**			
13	**Implements prescribed treatments in home**			
14	**Administers medications**			
	Oral			
	Parenteral			
	Intramuscular			
	Subcutaneous			
	Hypodermic			
	Intradermal			
	Assisting in intravenous infusions			
	Instillation of drops			
	Eye			
	Ear			
	Nose			
	Eye irrigation			
	Ear irrigation			
15	**Implements Community Health Nursing Process**			
16	**Maintains records, reports and registers**			
17	**Assists in conduction of special clinics**			
	MCH clinic			
	Antenatal clinic			
	Postnatal clinic			
	Under-five clinic			

Contd...

Contd...

Sl No	Name of the procedure	Date of demo	Date of return demonstration	Clinical Supervisor signature
	School health clinic			
	Family planning clinic			
	Geriatric clinic			
	Industrial clinic			
	Well baby clinic			
	Health camps			
	Assisting in safe motherhood and safe childhood activities			
18	**Assist in**			
	MCH activities			
	RCH program activities			
	Baby-friendly initiative activities			
	School health program activities			
	Industrial health program activities			
	Collect and calculate the vital statistics			
19	**Participates in prevention and control of communicable diseases**			
20	**Community health aspects of nutrition**			
a	Assess anthropometric measurements of children in home			
	Check and records Height			
	Weight			
	Head circumference			
	Mid-upper arm circumference			
	Chest circumference			
b	Educating community about nutrition			
	Nutrition deficiency disorders and its prevention			
	Prevention of food adulteration and its importance			
	Food and water sanitation			
	Preservation of food			
	Breastfeeding and weaning diet			

Contd...

Contd...

Sl No	Name of the procedure	Date of demo	Date of return demonstration	Clinical Supervisor signature
c	Assisting in implementation of National nutritional program activities			
	Nutritional rehabilitation activities			
	National days			
d	Supplements the child (under 3 year of age) with vitamin A solution			
21	**Immunizes the focus group with specific vaccines (primary and booster doses)**			
	Maintains cold chain system			
22	**Carrying out health education activities**			
	Individual			
	Family			
	Group			
	Mass			
	Preparation and effectively utilizes appropriate audio-visual aids during health education activities			
23	**Assists in empowerment for self-care of individuals, families and groups**			
24	**Assisting health professionals in carrying out health related activities within the community**			
25	**Utilizes techniques of supervision in monitoring health related activities**			
26	**Maintains good working relationship among health team members**			
27	**Prepares evaluation tools**			
28	**Document and maintain individual, family and administrative records, reports and registers**			
29	**Assists in**			
	Staff development programs			
	Inservice education programs			
	Continuing education programs			
	Skill training programs			
	Project work/research activities			
	Individual			
	Group			

Contd...

Contd...

Sl No	Name of the procedure	Date of demo	Date of return demonstration	Clinical Supervisor signature
30	**Assists in out reach program activities**			
31	**Assists in implementation of family welfare services**			
	Maintaining eligible couple register			
	Assists in insertion of IUD			
	Educating the eligible couple and community about Advantages and disadvantages of FP Methods			
	Adverse effects of population explosion			
32	**Counsel and teach individual, family and community about**			
	HIV, TB, DM, HTN			
	Adolescents' and elderly's health			
	Maintainance the health of physically, mentally challenged individuals			
33	**Utilizes community resources for self and family**			
	Trauma services			
	Old age homes			
	Orphanages			
	Homes for physically and mentally challenged individuals			
	Homes for destitutes			

Observational Visits

Sl No.	Place of visit	Date	Clinical Supervisor signature
1	Health organization		
2	MCH clinic		
3	RCH training center		
4	School		
5	Rural health center		
6	Local industries		
7	Rehabilitation homes		
8	Waste management units		

Family Study/Family Profile

Sl No	Family study	Date of presentation	Clinical Supervisor signature
1			
2			
3			

Family Care Plans

Sl No	Family care plan	Date of submission	Clinical Supervisor signature
1			
2			
3			

Ward Teaching Classes

Sl No	Topic	Date of presentation	Signature of Supervisor
1			
2			
3			
4			
5			

Health Education Activities

Sl No	Topic	Type of AV aids used	Place of presentation	Focus group	Date of presentation	Clinical Supervisor signature
1						
2						
3						
4						
5						

Signature of the Class Coordinator
Date:

Signature of the Principal
Date:

MANAGEMENT OF NURSING SERVICES

Sl No	Clinical activity	Date of performance	Clinical Supervisor's signature
1	**Applies principles of management in rendering comprehensive nursing services**		
2	**Follows line of authority in implementing the activities**		
3	**Prepares organizational chart of hospital Nursing Service Department and Nursing Educational Institution**		
4	**Maintains policies and protocols of the hospital**		
5	**Draws physical lay out of Hospital and Nursing Educational institution**		
6	**Lists out the job responsibilities of hospital staff** – Nursing superintendent		
	– Head nurse		
	– Staff nurse		
	– Nursing aid		
7	**Prepares job responsibilities of Principal and Faculty of School of Nursing**		
8	**Prepares job responsibilities of Principal and Faculty of College of Nursing**		
9	**Maintains leadership styles based on situation**		
10	**Maintains and checks inventory registers** – Supplies		
	– Equipment		
	– Linen		
	– Drugs		
11	**Distributes diet according to disease condition and as per doctor's order**		
12	**Maintains records and reports in the hospital** – Census		
	– Admission register		
	– Discharge register		
	– Dhobi register		
	– Equipment register		
	– Supplies register		
	– Indent register		
	– Birth register		
	– Death register		

Contd...

Contd...

Sl No	Clinical activity	Date of performance	Clinical Supervisor's signature
	Drug indent		
	Condemnation of equipments register		
	Register for narcotic drugs		
	Client files		
	Nurses round book		
	Doctors round book		
	Lab register		
	CSSD register		
	Nurses report		
	Morning		
	Evening		
	Night		
	Kardex		
	Observes the records and reports maintained in the school		
	Observes the activities in Nursing Superintendent's office		
	Follows biomedical waste management		
	Triage application in emergency situation		
	Conducts small type of project works		
13	**Observes supervision**		
	Faculty/staff		
	Students		
	Class D employees		
14	**Preparation of duty rosters**		
	Mess		
	Clinicals		
	Hostel work		
	Supporting staff		
15	**Utilizes nursing service personnel in the clinical area for nursing education services**		
16	**Prepares evaluation tools**		
17	**Assists in organizing**		
	Staff development program		
	Inservice training program		
	Staff welfare program activities		

Contd...

Contd...

Sl No	Clinical activity	Date of performance	Clinical Supervisor's signature
	Continuing education program		
	Orientation training program		
	Skill training program		
18	**Participates in team nursing activities**		
19	**Reporting during shift change**		
20	**Follows doctors, nurses rounds**		
21	**Participates in clinical teaching**		
	Management of personnel		
	Patient assignment		
	Special assignment		
	Orients new professional to Work schedule		
	Clients		
	Job routine		
	Participates in Team nursing		
	Primary nursing		
22	**Observes the records maintained in School of Nursing and College of Nursing**		

Observational Visits

Sl No	Place of visit	Date	Signature of Clinical Supervisor
1	**Nursing Institutions**		
	School of Nursing		
	Government		
	Private		
	Colleges of Nursing		
	Government		
	Private		
2	**Professional bodies**		
	INC		
	TNAI		
	State Nursing Council		
3	**Voluntary organizations**		
	National		
	International		
4	**Hospital set-up**		
	Government		
	Private		

Signature of the Class Coordinator
Date:

Signature of the Principal
Date:

INTRODUCTION TO NURSING RESEARCH

Sl No	Research activities	Date	Clinical Supervisor signature
1	**Utilizes steps in research process while conducting project works and implements it in report writing**		
	Introduction		
	Background of the study		
	Need for the study		
	Statement of the problem		
	Objectives of the study		
	Operational definitions		
	Variables		
	Assumptions		
	Limitations		
	Hypothesis		
	Conceptual framework		
	Organization of the report		
	Review of related literature		
	Methodology		
	Research approach		
	Research design		
	Setting of the study		
	Statement of objectives		
	Setting of the study		
	Population		
	Sampling technique and size		
	Inclusion and exclusion criteria		
	Content validity		
	Development and description of the tool		
	Reliability		
	Pilot study		
	Data collection		
	Plan for data analysis		
	Applies statistical methods in description of findings		
	Descriptive statistics		
	Inferential statistics		
	Discussion of findings		

Contd...

Contd...

Sl No	Research activities	Date	Clinical Supervisor signature
	Summary and conclusion		
	Implications and recommendations		
	Bibliography and annexures		
2	**Assists in clinical research activities**		
3	**Uses different data collection techniques in gathering information**		
	Questionnaire		
	Interview schedule		
	Observation method		
	Data analysis and measurement		

Signature of the Class Coordinator
Date:

Signature of the Principal
Date:

NURSING EDUCATION

Sl No	Student activity	Date of performance	Supervisor signature
1	**Utilizes different philosophies knowledge in Nursing**		
2	**Prepares objectives based on blooms' classification**		
3	**Follows principles of teaching in teaching-learning process**		
4	**Performs the role of a teacher**		
5	**Preparation of rotation plans**		
	Individual rotation plan		
	Master rotation plan		
	Clinical rotation plan		
6	**Preparation and utilization of audio-visual aids in** Nursing education activities		
	Audio-aids		
	Visual-aids		
	Projected		
	Non-projected		
7	**Prepares** Course plan		
	Unit plan		
	Lesson plan		
8	**Plans assignments for the students**		
9	**Assists in** Organization of clinical experiences		
	Maintenance of records (teaching and learning)		
10	**Utilizes teaching methods in practice teaching classes**		
	Lecture method		
	Demonstration method		
	Discussion method		
	Questioning technique		
	Role play		
	Laboratory method		
	Project method		
	Seminar presentation		
	Problem-solving method		

Contd...

Contd...

Sl No	Student activity	Date of performance	Supervisor signature
	Simulation technique		
	Participates in team teaching		
	Utilizes clinical teaching methods – Nursing clinics		
	– Nursing rounds		
	– Nursing conferences		
	– Process recording		
	– Field trips		
	– Observational visits		
11	**Prepares evaluation tools** • Clinical performance tools		
	– Checklist		
	– Rating scale		
	• Classroom test		
	– Constructs test and administers for a group of students		
	– Objective type of items		
	– Subjective type of items		

Observational Visits

Sl No	Place of visit	Date	Signature of Supervisor
1	School of Nursing		
2	College of Nursing		
3	Educational Centers		
4	Libraries		

Signature of the Class Coordinator
Date:

Signature of the Principal
Date:

Internship (Integrated Practice)

Name of the Student ....
Reg. No. ....

Total Hours: 1750

Sl No	Subjects	Clinical Hours	Clinical Hours in Weeks	Signature of the Clinical Supervisor
1	Midwifery and Obstetrical Nursing	240	5	
2	Community Health Nursing—II	195	4	
3	Medical-Surgical Nursing (Adult and Geriatrics)	430	09	
4	Child Health Nursing	145	03	
5	Mental Health Nursing	95	02	
6	Research project	45	01	
	Total Hours	**1150**	**24**	

Note :

- Internship has to be carried out as 8 hours/day, 48 hours/week under supervised nursing practice
- 2 weeks of evening and night shift duties
- Fourth year final examination to be held only after completing internship
- Students will be supervised by nursing teachers during internship
- Total hours (IV Year = 600; internship = 1150) = 1750 hours.

CLINICAL EXPERIENCES DURING INTERNSHIP

Midwifery and Obstetrical Nursing

Total Weeks = 5 weeks

Areas	Duration (weeks)	Objectives	Skills to be Developed	Assignments	Signature of Clinical Supervisor
Labor Ward	2	Provide comprehensive care to mothers and neonates	Integrated Practice	Completion of essential requirements	
Neonatal Intensive Care Unit (NICU)	1				
Antenatal Experience	2			Case book recordings	

Community Health Nursing—II

Total Weeks = 4 weeks

Areas	Duration (weeks)	Objectives	Skills to be Developed	Assignments	Signature of Clinical Supervisor
Urban and Rural	4	Provide comprehensive care to individual, family and community	Integrated Group Practice	Group Project 1 – Rural 1 – Urban • Assess clinical performance with rating scale • Evaluation of project	

Medical-Surgical Nursing (Adult and Geriatrics)

Total Weeks = 9 weeks

Areas	Duration (weeks)	Objectives	Skills to be Developed	Assignments	Signature of Clinical Supervisor
Medical Ward	2	Provides comprehensive care to patients with medical-surgical conditions including emergencies	Integrated Practice	Assess clinical performance with rating scale	
Surgical Ward	2				
Critical Care Unit (ICCU)	1				
Casualty/ Emergency	2				
Operation Theater (Eye, ENT, Neuro)	2	Assist with common surgical operations			

Child Health Nursing

Total Weeks = 3 weeks

Areas	Duration (weeks)	Objectives	Skills to be developed	Assignments	Signature of clinical Supervisor
Pediatric Medical Ward (ICU)	1	Provide comprehensive care to children with medical conditions	Integrated Practice	Assess clinical performance with rating scale	
Pediatric Surgical Ward (ICU)	1	Provide comprehensive care to children with surgical conditions	Integrated Practice	Assess clinical performance with rating scale	
NICU	1	Provide intensive care to neonates	Integrated Practice	Assess clinical performance with rating scale	

Mental Health Nursing

Total Weeks = 2 weeks

Areas	Duration (weeks)	Objectives	Skills to be developed	Assignments	Signature of Clinical Supervisor
Psychiatry Ward	2	Provide comprehensive care to patients with mental health problems	Integrated Practice	Assess clinical performance with rating scale	

Practical Examination—IV Year

1. **Midwifery and Obstetrical Nursing—II**

Signature of

Internal Examiner Date:

External Examiner Date:

Supplementary Examination

Signature of

Internal Examiner Date:

External Examiner Date:

2. **Community Health Nursing—II**

Signature of

Internal Examiner Date:

External Examiner Date:

Supplementary Examination

Signature of

Internal Examiner Date:

External Examiner Date: